Why, What & How

Why, What & How

THE 3 MOST IMPORTANT QUESTIONS OF OUR WEIGHT LOSS & FITNESS JOURNEY

Arthur Taylor

ISBN: 1534833889
ISBN 13: 9781534833883

Table of Contents

Dedication

I would like to dedicate this series of books to my wife, Clarissa. She is an amazing woman who inspires me daily to be better than my best. I love you...
I would also like to Thank Kim Beard, for she is the one that helped me to create a path for my desire to help others many years ago. She is by far the most dedicated and inspirational trainer in the fitness world that anyone could be blessed to meet!!!
And I also want to Thank God. For creating in me a deep desire to help others and blessing me with the ability to do just that...

Introduction

So, you want to get fit, healthy, strong, powerful, lean and sexy? Well, these are just some reasons we hire Personal Trainers everyday. Other reasons could be to build our confidence, stamina, social interaction, our self worth and/or simply finding a date for the weekend. Sounds silly, but the truth is, we all have a reason and those reasons can and do vary.

As many of us know, the easiest way to find a solution to our need is to join a local gym. So we go and take the tour, we fill out the membership form and the dreaded financial automatic draft form. But we feel good! We are happy, as we just took the first step towards the better us. So we are all set. We have our workout cloths, our tennis shoes and water bottle. Not long into our workout, a gym employee comes over to us and introduces himself or herself as a Personal Trainer. They ask why we joined the gym and just by coincidence there is a special on training sessions. Usually it is 3-5 sessions for free and then if we want more we have to pay. But we are excited and we agree to the free ones. So off we go to fill out some more paperwork. They tell us that we can cancel if we don't want the sessions to continue, but what they don't tell us is it will take an act of Congress to do so.

Does any of this sound familiar? If so, you know that once the free sessions are done, you feel more lost than you did when you started. That is because that trainer, who has your best interest in mind, works on commission. They are not going to give you the full picture, the method of the madness, of your training so you have to be dependent upon them in order to progress. When in reality they are there to empower and teach you how to progress on your own after a relatively short period of time. So you either continue to pay for someone you can't always afford, or you get confused and lost in the gym which usually means you don't enjoy going and eventually give up and stop going. Simply to go back to doing the same things that you were doing before joining the gym. Only now they have your permission to charge you every month for a membership you aren't even using. Does the gym care? Are they calling you to see how you are doing because they miss seeing your face? No! Truth is, they could care less if you ever come back. They got your money and because you signed the annual contract your stuck. They know that based on research the average person joining a gym will be done and over it within 90 days. That means they get the next 9 months of your money for free!

Don't get me wrong, I am not bashing nor trying to tarnish trainers or gyms. Trainers are needed and necessary in many ways. However, there are many things you can learn to help yourself. There is an old saying that says, "It is not what you do for a person, but what you teach that person to do for their self, that makes them successful." And as far as gyms go, they have their operational methods and after all, business is business.

In this first book, I am going to teach you how you can do many of the things a trainer can do for you. My goal is to empower you with the knowledge that will set you up for individual success. After all, the only reason you should hire a trainer is because you want one, not because you need one.

CHAPTER 1

Knowing Our Why And How

Okay, great to have you with me on our journey!! One of the biggest questions many of us have once we decide to get into better shape is, "Where do I begin?" There are two common answers to this question. They are, "I must eat less." And/or "I must start walking or exercising." While both of those answers are good, it isn't quite the beginning.

The *true* beginning is to know our WHY. And not just the why as to why we want to be in better shape, but also the why as to how we got to be in the shape we are in right now. The answer to that question is very important. Matter of fact, it is the MOST important part of our whole training program! For if we don't understand our WHY, we will most likely return to this very spot once again. So our learning begins now. I want us to get a piece of paper and get ready to write. Got it? Ready? Let's go...

Now we are going to number the paper 1-10. Now we are going to write down as many WHY reasons we can think of. Give me a second so I can write mine...done? Okay, so some of us have written one thing and others have written twelve. That is fine. Some of us have more reasons then the rest. Now let us review our list. Many of us have put down the following:

1. I was always called fat and/or big boned.
2. Almost everyone in my family is fat, so it must be genetic.
3. Having children destroyed my body!
4. Due to an injury, I am not as active as I once was.
5. Life is crazy and I don't know how to eat right, let alone have time to exercise!

Truth is, there can be, and are, many whys. Not all of us have just one! But, as I stated, we must know our *WHY* before we can learn the *HOW*. A great deal like financial debt. Until we know *WHY* we overspend the way we do, we will probably always be in debt, i.e. spending more than we make, shopping for happiness, or keeping up with the Jones (by the way, they're broke too). Once we know our *WHY* we're in debt then we can focus on the *HOW*, how to change the behavior. So we get out of debt and manage our money better.

Same with our weight and physical condition, once we know *why* we are in "physical debt" per say, we can be receptive and open to learning the *HOW*. How is more enjoyable then the *WHY*! I get excited every time I learn a *how* because that means I am going to learn something that will change my life forever!! As long as I apply it...

Now that we have learned our *WHY*, let us begin to understand the *HOW*. Are you excited?!? I am too!!!

HOW we are going to get in better shape is through knowledge, and learning how to apply it. So here are the things we are going to need to know:

1. What is a Calorie?
2. What is a RMR/BMR?
3. What is an Expenditure Rate?
4. What is Lean Mass vs. Body Fat?
5. What is a Caloric Deficit?
6. What's next?

In the following chapters we will learn the answers to these questions, and how we can begin to apply them. Are you ready...LET'S GO!!!!!

CHAPTER 2

What Is A Calorie?

Welcome to Chapter 2! As you can already tell, I am not going to fill these pages with a bunch of quotes and confusing jargon. I am not here to write about everything I know of fitness and nutrition, hoping that you are so wowed with my depth of knowledge that you are impressed and mind blown. That would only lead to you reading a book that you may, or may not, completely understand and therefore makes it pointless. I am not the best trainer in the world nor is this going to be the very best book ever; after all, it is the very first book I have ever written. That being said, I am going to keep it simple, yet factual, so that no matter who picks this up to read will be able to completely grasp the concepts inside and be able to apply it to their everyday life. I want this book to be used as a knowledgeable tool, not as a paperweight or used storage on whatever device you used to download it. So let's get at it...

What is a calorie? A calorie is simply a unit of measurement. What is measured? Energy. Someone just said "What?" Let's learn. Without going into the deep end of the pool, there are two types of calories. There are small calories and large calories. Regardless of the size of the calorie, they both react the same. When a calorie is "broken down" it gives off heat. Heat is nothing more then energy that has been released. Based on how much heat is generated depends on how much energy is measured. That makes sense, right? Think about how we begin to sweat when we are physically active. We sweat due to the amount of calories we are using, and hence the heat that is being created. The body must cool itself and release that heat through our pores when it is excessive. Otherwise, we would boil from the inside...not good! Now we know what a calorie is. Why is that important?

It is important because we need calories to survive. Everything that our bodies do requires energy. From breathing, hearts beating, brains thinking to walking, talking and digesting our foods. On the same note, too many calories can kill us. Too many calories creates large deposits of fat, increases our blood pressure, screws up our hormones and ages us faster than we should, just to name a few. The key is to pinpoint the proper amount of calories we need to accomplish our goal of loosing unwanted weight or gaining some desired muscle, or both.

Are all calories created equal? Yes. As a matter of fact they are. Small calories are always small and large calories are always large. And as we learned a second ago, they both react in the same exact way. The key is, not all *foods* are created equal! Some foods have more calories than others, making them more caloric dense. Some examples are fats and oils, nuts and seeds, dried fruits and red meats. Other foods are not as calorie rich, or dense. Such as broccoli, apples, asparagus and fish. Individually none of these foods are bad for us. It is the frequency and the amounts we eat that create the negative and unwanted effects.

See, our bodies need a certain amount of calories per day in order to maintain our daily functions and repair any damage it might receive. Too many calories and our bodies store them as fat. Basically it's energy in the bank for a rainy day. Too little calories and our bodies hang on to them, storing them as fat, just in case it doesn't get enough energy tomorrow. So much of our problem is inconsistency. Some days we eat enough, others too much and yet other days not enough. So we inadvertently train our bodies to store fat and it has become extremely efficient at doing so. However, if we learn, and we will, how to give our bodies the proper amount of calories on a consistent daily basis, there will be no reason for it to store anything. Then we can begin working on burning that stored energy, and reducing the stored unwanted and undesirable fat.

That leads us into our next chapter, *What is my RMR/BMR*. In that chapter we will learn how to find out how many calories we need on a daily basis to maintain what we have right now.

Congratulations on learning what a calorie is!!! There is much more we can discuss about calories, but again, lets learn the very basics, build our foundation. We can, and will, learn more about them later. Chapter 3 is next...LET'S GO.

CHAPTER 3

What Is My RMR/BMR?

O ur journey continues and we find ourselves here at Chapter 3. Here we're going to learn about another *what* and then another *how*. I can feel the knowledge beginning to percolate up under my feet already and I am super excited!! Let's dive in...

Before we find our RMR or BMR, we must know what they are. RMR is short for *Resting Metabolic Rate*, while BMR is short for *Basal Metabolic Rate*. Both are ways of measuring (or estimating) the amount of calories we will burn while at rest over a 24-hour period.

So, picture sitting on a beach watching the seagulls fly and listening to the waves break on the shoreline. We sit there for 24-hours, but don't get up. Now, even though we are just sitting there, much is still going on. Our hearts are beating, lungs are breathing, and eyes are blinking. Our liver and kidneys are filtering and new skin, hair and nails are growing! And that isn't even all. As we learned in Chapter 2, all of these things require what? That's right, CALORIES! That is a good analogy of what our RMR is all about. Our BMR is similar, but much more difficult to gauge so it is done in a very strict medical lab or clinic.

Now, let's say we got up from where we are sitting and took a walk down the beach and back. Would that change anything? For sure it would! For as we now know, walking requires calories too; therefore we just burned calories while we were walking. Now we have what is called our Expenditure Rate. But we'll hold on to that for right now. We need to get through this chapter first and we'll learn about our Expenditure Rate (ER) in Chapter 4.

Okay. We now have an understanding about what a RMR and a BMR is. So let us begin to learn the *how* of our *what*.

In order to know what our RMR/BMR is, there are several different equations that measures the amount of calories burned per minute. Then you multiply by 1,440 to find the total calories burned over a 24-hour period. This equation is often used in conjunction with indirect calosimetry, which uses spent gases to calculate the type and amount of gases we are utilizing. It looks like this:

$$REE=[3.9(VO2)+1.1(VCO2)]\ 1.44$$

VO2 is the amount, or volume, of oxygen we breathe in (mL/min) per minute. VCO2 is the amount, or volume, of carbon dioxide we breathe out (mL/min) per minute. This gives us our "Respiratory Quotient".

$$RQ=VCO2/VO2$$

Our BMR is much more intricate and difficult, as stated earlier. It involves our RMR, our thermogenic effect of food (TEF), our non-exercise activity thermogenesis (NEAT), excess post-exercise oxygen consumption (EPOC), and exercise (EX). All of this put together will give us our total daily energy expenditure (TDEE). But let us not stress or worry, for to properly calculate that accurately we need a clinic setting with doctors that know how to do it.

I told you I would not get too technical and jargonize stuff and I won't. I just wanted us to see how difficult this stuff is to learn at times. And we are going to learn a much easier way to find that stuff out! So let us get back to the way we can find this information out for ourselves.

That place is....the internet! There are several links on every search engine that we can simply plug in some numbers and with relative accuracy find our RMR/BMR. I am not going to recommend any particular search engine, or site, to use for I am not going to endorse or suggest one over another. If I did, I would have to create a cite list in the back of this book and honestly, I don't want to do that. After all, nobody is going to read that page...

So, we go to our search engine and type in "RMR Calculator". Any of the first 3 is great as those are usually the most used. Click on one and somewhere on the page it will ask us for our age, gender, height and weight. We punch in those numbers, click on "calculate" (or submit), and BOOM, there is our RMR! Easy enough, right?

Now that we have our RMR, what do we do with it? The answer is, nothing for now. We'll write it down so we don't forget it and we will use it here in a bit.

This is exciting! Now we know what a calorie is and why it is important. We know what a RMR and BMR is *and* we know how to find out what ours is. Which means we now know how many calories we need to stay alive if we were to just relax for 24-hours. Next we are going to learn what an Expenditure Rate (ER) is *and*, you got it, *how* to find out ours. We are learning a good deal and it is said that knowledge is power. We are feeling more and more confident and self sufficient with every chapter so lets continue...On to the next chapter!

CHAPTER 4

What Is An Expenditure Rate (ER)?

Remember in Chapter 3 we had the analogy of sitting on the beach relaxing? Then we went for a walk and we called that our Expenditure Rate? Well we are going to look at that a bit more now.

An *Expenditure Rate* (ER) is simply the amount, or number, of calories we burn while in motion or doing an activity. As we know, calories are required for everything we do while alive. So let us continue with using that analogy for the following example. Here goes...

We are going to say that simply sitting there on the beach gives us a RMR of 2000 calories. So, in order for us to function in our current condition we are using 200 calories per day. The next day we get up and go for that walk down the beach and back. We're going to say that burned 500 more calories. The 500 calories is our ER. *NOW*, in order to stay alive in our current condition, we need to consume 2500 calories per day.

$$RMR+ER=daily\ caloric\ need$$

There is another equation called the "Harris Benedict Formula" that is commonly used to find our daily caloric needs. I am not going to write it out for us, for we can do it simpler and quicker another way.

Just as we found our RMR/BMR by using the search engine, we can also find out our daily caloric need the same way. We would go to our search engine and type in "daily caloric needs calculator" in do as we did before. Punch in our numbers, and

BOOM, there we have it. But here is another way we can do it. We take our RMR/BMR, remember we wrote that down for later, and multiply it by one of the following:

- 1.2 (if we are not exercising)
- 1.375 (if we are exercising lightly, say 1-3 times a week)
- 1.55 (if we are exercising moderately, say 3-5 times per week)
- 1.725 (if we are exercising hard, say 6-7 days per week)
- 1.9 (if we are going crazy and exercising extremely hard, say 6-7 days a week plus working construction or something)

Okay, now, using the number we used earlier, let us say that our RMR/BMR is 2000 and we are going to exercise 3-5 days per week. So we multiply our 2000 calories by 1.55.

$$2000 \times 1.55 = 3100 \text{ calories}$$

Now in order to stay alive in the condition we are in we need 3100 calories per day. We have now found the sweet spot! Now we know how many calories our body requires in order for it to stop storing calories as fat. All we have to do is simply eat them and we're good. We're not eating too many, nor are we eating too little, we're eating just right! And we have to eat them consistently.

But what if we want to loose that unwanted and undesirable fat? Or what if we wanted to put on some muscle? Or both? Well, before we can properly do that we need to find out how much fat and muscle we currently have. And we are going to learn how to find those answers in the next chapter.

To review, we have learned the following already:

1. What a calorie is and why it is important
2. What a RMR/BMR is and how to find ours
3. What an Expenditure Rate is and how to get ours
4. How many calories we need to consume per day in order for our body to not store anymore unwanted fat.

Next we are going to learn about body fat and lean mass. After we know the *what*, we will learn the *how* of finding ours. Let us continue...

CHAPTER 5

What Is Body Fat & Lean Mass?

Body Fat (BF) and Lean Mass (LM) are the things that that make up our weight. We'll begin with our BF and then we will hit our LM, and we will learn how to find our numbers.

Body Fat is exactly what it sounds like. Fat. But there are different types of fat and different functions for each. Let's learn about them.

There is *Brown* fat, which when stimulated, can burn calories. Lean people tend to have more of this fat than overweight people. Brown fat is found primarily in children, and begins to decline, as they get older. When Brown fat is stimulated, it burns White fat.

White fat is the most common of fats. Even though leaner people have more Brown fat, every one of us has more White fat by far. White fat is used to store energy and produce hormones. One of the pluses of White fat is that it produces a hormone called *adiponectin*. That hormone makes our liver and muscles more sensitive to *insulin*, another hormone, which makes us less susceptible to diabetes and heart disease. But, too much White fat causes that production to slow way down or even stop altogether. Leading us closer to those diseases.

Then there is *Subcutaneous* fat. This is found directly under our skin. This fat isn't as dangerous as once believed, unless it is located in the dreaded belly area! For that is when it is tied into our visceral fat.

Visceral fat is fat that is coating or wrapped around our internal organs, like our liver and stomach, intestines and our heart. Visceral fat is nasty stuff!!! It shoots our risk of heart disease, diabetes, strokes and dementia through the ozone. Not to mention it leaks toxins into our blood stream!

So, as we can see, we all have the same types of fat. The difference is some of us have more or less of them all. It is also interesting to note that we are all born with a certain number of fat cells. As we get older that number neither increases nor decreases. That is because fat is an organ. We may wonder, "then why do we put on fat?" Here is our answer. Fat cells are like little sacks. When our body begins to store energy, excess calories, it goes to our fat cells and begins to fill them up. Causing them to expand. When we loose fat, the opposite happens. The fat is released into our bloodstream through a hormonal process and the cells are emptied and become smaller. It has been proven that people that get "lipo Suction", which removes fat cells from the body, regenerate those cells back within a 4 years period on average. So don't waste your hard earned money!!!

Those are the basics of fats, so let us move on to Lean Mass...

Lean Mass (LM) is everything else that our bodies are comprised of. From our hair, nails, teeth, bones, muscles and organs, etc. What we are concerned about is our muscles. Though everything else is extremely important, our muscles burn more calories than anything else. They are our body's caloric furnace per say. So, the more muscle we have, the more calories we will use and the leaner we will become.

Just as there are various types of BF there are various types of muscles. There is *Cardiac*, found only around our heart. There is *Skeletal*, which helps move our joints and bones. And, there is *Smooth* muscle, which is what forms our organs, like our bladder and stomach. We are going to concern ourselves with skeletal muscle. There isn't much of anything we can do to increase our LM in the Cardiac or Smooth muscle area, though we can strengthen them through cardio exercise and resistant training. But we'll get there later...

In this book we are not going to get into the anatomy of these things, or into our energy pathways or hormone processes. We don't need, nor are we ready, for that type of information yet. We will however, briefly cover the types of skeletal muscles so we understand a bit more about them.

There are three types of skeletal muscles:

1. Slow Twitch Fibers (Type 1): These are our endurance muscles. They typically contract slowly and can continue to do so over a long period of time before tiring. They are smaller and less powerful than fast twitch fibers. We use these

muscles in activities such as walking or folding cloths. They are "red" fibers, as they require oxygen to function properly.

2. Fast Twitch Fibers (Type 2a): These are much faster muscles compare to our Type 1 muscles. These are "white" fibers as they are not as reliant on oxygen to function; therefore they also tire much more rapidly. Activities using these muscle fibers are weight training with moderate reps and running down the block.

3. Fast Twitch Fibers (Type 2b): These are our fastest muscles! They are white like the Type 2a but are different as they are only used without oxygen, and tire much quicker due to that. Activities using these fibers are sprints, power lifting and heavy weight lifting (1-3 reps).

I know we got somewhat technical with muscles and fats but I wanted you to get an idea of what we are working with. In our next book we will go further into the subject by covering the muscles and fats in the areas of genetics, blood hormone levels, training and variations by population to mention a few. It is going to be fun as it is all very informative!!

So, we now know our *what* of LM and BF. Now we'll learn *how* to find our numbers. First we need a regular flexible tape measure. Once we have our tapes we are going to take some basic measurements. All of which we can do ourselves with relative ease. We are going to measure the following:

- Waist (at our belly button)
- Right wrist*
- Hips (at the widest part of our butt)*
- Right forearm (the thickest part)*

The * indicates for women only. Guys just need the waist measurement. Now we are going TO THE SEARCH ENGINE! We're going to type in "Body Fat Calculator" and pick on of the top three, just as we did before to find our RMR/BMR. Now we are going to type in our info. We see we need our gender and weight. We also need our waist, wrist, hip and forearm measurements. Depending on preference and/or location, do inches or metric. Now we hit calculate and BOOM we have our BF%.

Now to find our LM we go back to our search engine and type in "Lean Mass Calculator". Once there we will type in our weight and BF%, clicks calculate and

BOOM, we now know our LM. Now, we take our LM and subtract that from our current weight and we knowhow much fat we have in pounds.

For example: If we weigh 200 pounds and our BF% is 40%, our LM would be 120 pounds. We subtract 200-120=80. So we now know we have 120 pounds of LM and 80 pounds of fat. Now, if we desire to weigh 140 pounds we need to lose 60 pounds of BF. In Chapter 6 we will learn what a *Caloric Deficit* is and how to create ours.

So lets go there now...

CHAPTER 6

What Is A Caloric Deficit And What Comes Next?

n this final chapter we will cover the last two questions. We're almost done, so lets dive in...

What is a Caloric Deficit? Simply put, it is the number of calories we eat less than the calories required for our RMR/BMR and ER. An example would be if our calculated RMR was 2000 calories and our ER was 500 calories, our required caloric intake for the day would be 2500 calories (remember our example in Chapter 3). But, if we only eat 2000 calories, we have created a CD of 500 calories. The cool thing is this, 3500 calories make up one pound of body fat. So, if we create a CD of 500 calories for one week, 7 days, we will have lost one pound of BF! Pretty awesome right!! Who knew it could be so easy!!! We can also create a CD by exercising. Remember in our example (Chapter 3) we burned calories by walking down the beach. So if we eat 500 calories less and we burn 500 calories by exercising, that is a CD of 1000 calories per day. That is 7000 calories per week, which is two pounds of BF lost!!! (The opposite is needed to create muscle. We add 500 calories per day giving us a caloric surplus of 3500 calories per week.)

Now we know what a CD is, and we know that there is not one, but two ways of creating it. So what's next? We are going to learn! Get ready, because we are now going to put it all together. And you will see just how easy and simple it is. Once we're done we will have our *what* and our *how*. We will have the powerful knowledge needed to begin making an immediate change in our lives forever. And not only can we use this power to change our lives, we can teach it to others we know and love. We are about to have the knowledge and power to change the world!

Here's **HOW** we do it...

1. We **MUST** understand our WHY!!! Again, this is the single most important part of it all. If we jump in without knowing our why we are doomed to fall back into the same spot we are in right now. So don't rush this part. Get that paper and make your list of whys. Get deep and personal with it, because it is often deep and personal! Were you bullied growing up because you were different? Were you abused mentally, emotionally, physically and/or sexually? Were you/are you in an unloving family or relationship? Have you become depressed and just are not active anymore? Have you had children and just don't seem to have the energy or time to get yourself back? Maybe an injury some time ago has created a pattern of sedentariness. Bottom line, there are quadrillion different whys, all valid and understandable and you need to find your and understand it. Never think you are on an island by yourself. Believe me, we all are struggling and want to be better tomorrow than we are today. To be honest and transparent with you, I was locked in a room for 7 years. I was physically, mentally, and emotionally and for the last 4 years of it, sexually abused by my stepmother. At one point my room was a hallway closet in which I had a beanbag as my bed. I was fed once or twice a day and was only let out to go to school each day. And guess what, NOBODY knew what was going on at home!! I was too afraid and I also thought that this was how everyone else lived, so why bother to talk about it. I could go deeper into it but I wanted to share that with you so that you can see, know and understand that we all have craziness in our lives that have helped to create our current situation, and once we know our why, we can begin to understand it and know that we have the power to change everything for the better! Sometimes professional help is needed to work through things and that is okay.

2. Finding our RMR/BMR. We know that we require calories to function and survive. But how many is different for us all. We know that the variances are in our height, weight, age, gender and current activity level. Now all we need to do is hit that search engine, type in RMR/BMR Calculator and click on any of the top three. Type in our numbers and BOOM.

3. Finding our Expenditure Rate (ER). Now we have our RMR/BMR number so all we need to do is multiply based on our activity level (refer to Chapter 4). Now we know how many calories we need per day to maintain our current

weight. If we are happy with where we are at, doubtful, we can just stop right here. Eat those calories each day and we are good. But we know we are not, so on to Step 4.

4. Finding our Body Fat and Lean Mass Percentages. We know what fat is, and we know what lean mass is. Now we will find out about how much of each we have. To the search engine! Type in Body Fat calculator and we are going to punch in our numbers and BOOM. Now we are going to do the same for our Lean Mass, for we must have our BF% before we can do this. Same process as with BF. Click on calculate and BOOM. We have our BF% and our LM.

5. Creating our Caloric Deficit. We know that a minus can be created by eating less than our daily needs and/or by adding exercise daily. Now we take our caloric needs number for the day and we eat 500 calories less. That will help us loose one pound per week. We also know that if we add exercise to our day we can possibly burn an additional 500 calories per day, creating a two pound lose per week, for 3500 calories equates to one pound of BF so doing both together we hit that 7000 calorie mark each week!

And we are on our way!!!!

Now we don't have to be lost, not knowing where to begin. Having to trust that someone else has our best interest in mind and will set us up for success. Wondering how to gather the information needed and how to piece it all together so it works. Because we all have now empowered ourselves! We have the knowledge we need and are ready to begin one of the most exciting new chapters in our lives. We have the ability, the desire, the determination and will. For we know our *WHY, WHAT* and *HOW!!!*

Summary

A s I mentioned in the Introduction (hope we all read that) this book is about simple knowledge needed to get us moving in the positive direction we desire to go, without the cost of a gym membership or training fees. It is not a quantity of info, but quality info! There is much more we need to know if we are going to take this to the next level, and we will learn that in book #2. We will continue to learn the information and steps needed, in digestible pieces, so that we don't become overwhelmed and frustrated. All the while becoming more powerful with the strength of our gain knowledge.

I want to **_THANK YOU_** for coming on this knowledge based journey of fat lose with me and as well, I desire to keep up with you on your personal journey. As you know, I am here to make things as easy and as understandable as possible. So send me your questions, comment and/or feedback. Send me your before and after pictures with your contact info (I do not post/share any pictures without written permission). If you have any ideas and/or suggestions about another book you haven't seen yet let me know, I will see about writing it.

Now, while you go get this started, I am going to begin writing Book #2 of our series and I'll be waiting to hear from you!

Love you ALL...

P.S. Always remember to get a doctor's okay before you begin ANY nutritional and/or daily activity program!!! Especially if you happen to be on any medications, have recently given birth (CONGTATS!!!) and/or are recovering from an injury/surgery as I am NOT a doctor and I can't give you that okay, okay?!?!

About me...

My name is Bruce and I have been a Personal Trainer/Nutritionist for close to two decades now. I have worked with clients as old as 4 and as young as 82. I have experience in a wide variety of areas, from Pre and Post Natal, Diabetes: Type 1 and 2, Bodybuilding/Fitness/Figure, Injury recovery, MMA, Strength and Endurance conditioning just to name a few. I have also had the honor and privilege of working with the USAF and USMC in helping our brave service members with their CFT, PFT and the BCP programs.

Along with nearly 20 years of experience, I am also a CFT, FS, ASFN. I am also AED/CPR Cert. as well as insured.

Whatever your fitness goal, I can help you achieve it !!!

Contact Info...

www.globalfitness.training
Bruce@globalfitness.training
1-(619) 200-5750